Sirtfood *Diet*

cookbook

FOR BEGINNERS

With Easy and Healthy Recipes for a Rapid Weight Loss Burn Your Fat and Improve Your Metabolism With The Sirt Foods

ASHLEY GOSLING

DEDICATION

This book is dedicated to everyone who wants to live a healthier lifestyle and challenge himself of herself with this noble purpose.
Every little success is a great success in reality.

Every little step matters.

TABLE OF CONTENTS

DISCLAIMER

All the informations included in this book are given for instructive, informational and entertainment purposes, the author can claim to share very good quality recipes but is not headed for the perfect data and uses of the mentioned recipes, in fact the informations are not intent to provide dietary advice without a medical consultancy.

The author does not hold any responsibility for errors, omissions or contrary interpretation of the content in this book.

It is recommended to consult a medical practitioner before to approach any kind of diet, especially if you have a particular health situation, the author isn't headed for the responsibility of these situations and everything is under the responsibility of the reader, the author strongly recommend to preserve the health taking all precautions to ensure ingredients are fully cooked.

All the trademarks and brands used in this book are only mentioned to clarify the sources of the informations and to describe better a topic. All the trademarks and brands mentioned own their copyrights and they are not related in any way to this document and to the author.

This document is written to clarify all the informations of publishing purposes and cover any possible issue. This document is under copyright and it is not possible to reproduce any part of this content in every kind of digital or printable document. All rights reserved.

Spinach Green Juice

Prep Time   10 min

Servings   1

INGREDIENTS

- 1 bunch spinach
- 1 kiwi fruit
- 1 apple
- large stalks green celery, including leaves
- half a lemon, juiced
- 1 tsp. matcha green tea

DIRECTIONS

1. Extract the juice of spinach, apple and kiwi fruit.
2. Pour a Half juice into a glass, then add the matcha, lemon juice and mix well with fork.
3. Once the matcha is dissolved add the
4. remainder of the juice.
5. Mix well.
6. Pour some water on top.
7. Enjoy!

NUTRITIONAL INFORMATION
Calories Per Servings, 181 kcal, 1.72 g Fat, 39.64 g Total Carbs, 10.41 g Protein, 12.2 g Fiber

Berries Green Juice

Prep Time   10 min
Servings   1

INGREDIENTS

- 1 bunch mint leaves
- 1 apple
- ¼ cup mix berries
- 1/8 tsp. ginger
- half a lemon, juiced
- 1 tsp. matcha green tea

DIRECTIONS

1. Extract the juice of mint leaves, apple and berries.
2. Pour a Half juice into a glass, then add the matcha, lemon juice and mix well with fork.
3. Once the matcha is dissolved add the
4. remainder of the juice.
5. Mix well.
6. Pour some water on top.
7. Enjoy!

NUTRITIONAL INFORMATION

Calories Per Servings, 121 kcal, 0.49 g Fat, 32.2 g Total Carbs, 0.85 g Protein, 5.3 g Fiber

Broccoli Green Juice

Prep Time   10 min

Servings   1

INGREDIENTS

- 1 bunch spinach
- 1 apple
- 1 cup broccoli
- 1/8 tsp ginger.
- half a lemon, juiced
- 1 tsp. matcha green tea

DIRECTIONS

1. Extract the juice of spinach, apple and broccoli florets.
2. Pour a Half juice into a glass, then add the matcha, lemon juice and mix well with fork.
3. Once the matcha is dissolved add the
4. remainder of the juice.
5. Mix well.
6. Pour some water on top.
7. Enjoy!

NUTRITIONAL INFORMATION

Calories Per Servings, 187 kcal, 1.89 g Fat, 40.33 g Total Carbs, 11.56 g Protein, 13 g Fiber

Mix Green Juice

Prep Time   10 min

Servings   1

INGREDIENTS
- 1 bunch parsley
- 1 apple
- 1 cucumber
- half a lemon, juiced
- 1 tsp. matcha green tea

DIRECTIONS

1. Extract the juice of parsley apple and cucumber.
2. Pour a Half juice into a glass, then add the matcha, lemon juice and mix well with fork.
3. Once the matcha is dissolved add the
4. remainder of the juice.
5. Mix well.
6. Pour some water on top.
7. Enjoy!

NUTRITIONAL INFORMATION

Calories Per Servings, 146 kcal, 1.16 g Fat, 33.93 g Total Carbs, 3.53 g Protein, 7.8 g Fiber

Celery Green Juice

Prep Time   10 min

Servings   1

INGREDIENTS

- 5 -8 stalks celery with leaves
- 1 apple
- half a lemon, juiced
- 1 tsp. matcha green tea

DIRECTIONS

1. Extract the juice of celery and apple.
2. Pour a Half juice into a glass, then add the matcha, lemon juice and mix well with fork.
3. Once the matcha is dissolved add the
4. remainder of the juice.
5. Mix well.
6. Pour some water on top.
7. Enjoy!

NUTRITIONAL INFORMATION

Calories Per Servings, 118 kcal, 0.55 g Fat, 3o.07 g Total Carbs, 1.33 g Protein, 6.2 g Fiber

Kale Green Juice

Prep Time   10 min

Servings   1

INGREDIENTS

- 2 bunch kale
- 1 apple
- 2 stalk celery with leaves
- half a lemon, juiced
- 1 tsp. matcha green tea

DIRECTIONS

1. Extract the juice of kale, apple and celery.
2. Pour a Half juice into a glass, then add the matcha, lemon juice and mix well with fork.
3. Once the matcha is dissolved add the
4. remainder of the juice.
5. Mix well.
6. Pour some water on top.

Enjoy!

NUTRITIONAL INFORMATION

Calories Per Servings, 171 kcal, 1.67 g Fat, 39.53 g Total Carbs, 6.54 g Protein, 9.8 g Fiber

Spinach & Apple Juice

Prep Time   10 min

Servings   1

INGREDIENTS

- 1 bunch baby spinach
- 1 apple
- half a lemon, juiced
- 1 tsp. matcha green tea

DIRECTIONS

1. Extract the juice of spinach, and apple.
2. Pour a Half juice into a glass, then add the matcha, lemon juice and mix well with fork.
3. Once the matcha is dissolved add the
4. remainder of the juice.
5. Mix well.
6. Pour some water on top.

Enjoy!

NUTRITIONAL INFORMATION

Calories Per Servings, 178 kcal, 1.69 g Fat, 39.13 g Total Carbs, 10.29 g Protein, 11.9 g Fiber

Cucumber Green Juice

Prep Time   10 min

Servings   1

INGREDIENTS

- 1 cucumber
- 1 green apple
- half a lemon, juiced
- 1 tsp. matcha green tea

DIRECTIONS

1. Extract the juice of cucumber and apple.
2. Pour a Half juice into a glass, then add the matcha, lemon juice and mix well with fork.
3. Once the matcha is dissolved add the
4. remainder of the juice.
5. Mix well.
6. Pour some water on top.

Enjoy!

NUTRITIONAL INFORMATION

Calories Per Servings, 124 kcal, 0.69 g Fat, 31.13 g Total Carbs, 1.75 g Protein, 5.8 g Fiber

Creamy Spinach Juice

Prep Time   10 min

Servings   1

INGREDIENTS

- 1 bunch spinach
- ½ cup soy milk
- half a medium green apple
- half a lemon, juiced
- 1 tsp. matcha green tea

DIRECTIONS

1. Extract the juice of spinach and apple.
2. Pour a Half juice into a glass, then add the matcha, lemon juice and mix well with fork.
3. Once the matcha is dissolved add the remainder of the juice.
4. Mix well.
5. Pour some water on top.
6. Enjoy!

NUTRITIONAL INFORMATION

Calories Per Servings, 185 kcal, 3.35 g Fat, 32.68 g Total Carbs, 13.28 g Protein, 10 g Fiber

Parsley Green Juice

Prep Time   10 min

Servings   1

INGREDIENTS

- 1 bunch parsley
- 1 apple
- large stalks green celery, including leaves
- half a lemon, juiced
- 1 tsp. matcha green tea

DIRECTIONS

Extract the juice of parsley apple and stalk.

1.   Pour a Half juice into a glass, then add the matcha, lemon juice and mix well with fork.
2.   Once the matcha is dissolved add the
3.   remainder of the juice.
4.   Mix well.
5.   Pour some water on top.
6.   Enjoy!

NUTRITIONAL INFORMATION

Calories Per Servings, 124 kcal, 0.87 g Fat, 31.9 g Total Carbs, 2.47 g Protein, 6.7 g Fiber

Apple Porridge

Prep Time   10 Min

Servings   4

INGREDIENTS

- 2 apples, chopped
- 3 cups walnut milk
- 1 tsp. cinnamon
- 2 tsp. dates syrup
- TOPPING
- Blueberries
- dark chocolate
- apple slice
- walnuts

DIRECTIONS

1. Mix all ingredients together in a bowl that fits inside the bowl of your slow cooker.
2. Place the bowl in your slow cooker, and fill your slow cooker with 1 cup of water to surround the bowl.

3. Cook on LOW 6-8 hours, stirring occasionally.
4. Carefully remove the bowl.
5. Top with banana slice and berries.
6. Serve and enjoy!

NUTRITIONAL INFORMATION

Calories Per Servings, 227 kcal, 7.04 g Fat, 36.45 g Total Carbs, 6.95 g Protein, 4.3 g Fiber

Spinach Omelet

Prep Time   20 min

Servings   2

INGREDIENTS

- 2 cups baby spinach, finely chopped
- 1 cup, chopped onion
- 1 cup buckwheat flour
- ¼ cup water
- salt & pepper to taste
- 1 tsp. paprika powder
- 1 tsp. oregano
- olive oil for frying

DIRECTIONS

1. Mix flour, spinach, salt, pepper, oregano and paprika in a bowl and mix well.
2. Add water slowly in the mixture to make a thick batter.
3. Place a frying pan over medium heat and grease with olive oil.
4. Pour ¼ cup mixture in skillet and spread it evenly.
5. Once cooked, flip and cook for another 2-3 minutes.

6. Once the omelet is cooked remove from heat.
7. Serve with spinach leaves, tomato slice, and cucumber slice.
8. Enjoy!

NUTRITIONAL INFORMATION

Calories Per Servings, 283 kcal, 3.02 g Fat, 57.39 g Total Carbs, 14.52 g Protein, 12.5 g Fiber

Tofu & Kale Toast

Prep Time   10 min

Servings   4

INGREDIENTS
- 1 tsp. capers, drained and loosely chopped
- sea salt and black pepper
- 1 tsp. sesame seeds
- 1/4 cup guacamole
- 8 oz. tofu, firm and drained
- 4 slices buckwheat bread
- 4 oz. kale
- 1 tbsp. olive oil

DIRECTIONS
1. Heat olive oil in pan over medium heat and fry tofu until golden brown from all sides.
2. Add capers, salt and pepper to a mixing bowl.
3. Taste and adjust seasonings as needed.
4. Toast bread on heated griddle for 2-3 minutes per side.
5. Spread guacamole on each bread slice and arrange in plate.
6. Arrange tofu on bread slice with kale.
7. Drizzle sesame seeds.
8. Serve and enjoy!

NUTRITIONAL INFORMATION

Calories Per Servings, 216 kcal, 17.36 g Fat, 8.43 g Total Carbs, 10.45 g Protein, 3.5 g Fiber

Tofu Scramble

Prep Time   20 min

Servings   2

INGREDIENTS
- 1 tablespoon olive oil
- 16 oz. block firm tofu
- 1 teaspoon salt
- 1/4 teaspoon turmeric
- 1/4 teaspoon garlic powder
- 2 tablespoons soy milk

DIRECTIONS
1.   Heat the olive oil in a pan over medium heat. Mash the block of tofu right in the pan, with a potato masher or a fork.
2.   Cook, stirring frequently, for 3-4 minutes until the water from the tofu is dried.
3.   Add salt, turmeric and garlic powder. Cook and stir constantly for about 5 minutes.
4.   Pour the milk into the pan, and stir to mix. Serve immediately.
5.Enjoy!

NUTRITIONAL INFORMATION

Calories Per Servings, 208 kcal, 15.44 g Fat, 5.45g Total Carbs, 15.2 g Protein, 0.6 g Fiber

Buckwheat Pancakes

Prep Time   20 min

Servings   3

INGREDIENTS

- 1 cup buckwheat flour
- 2 tbsps. dates syrup
- 1 cup soya milk
- 1 tbsps. olive oil

DIRECTIONS

1. Mix all ingredients in bowl.
2. Heat oil in pan over medium heat. Once oil is hot pour ¼ cup buckwheat batter and spread evenly.
3. Cook for 2-3 minutes until golden brown.
4. Flip and cook again.
5. Once cooked remove from heat.
6. Serve and enjoy!

NUTRITIONAL INFORMATION

Calories Per Servings, 197 kcal, 3.92 g Fat, 35.68 g Total Carbs, 7.73 g Protein, 4.43g Fiber

Waffle Sandwich

Prep Time   10 min

Servings   4

INGREDIENTS
- 1 1/2 cups buckwheat flour
- 2 teaspoons baking powder
- 1 teaspoon baking soda
- 1/4 teaspoon salt
- 1/4 teaspoon cinnamon, optional
- 1 1/2 cups soy milk,
- 1 tablespoon apple cider vinegar
- 1/8 cup olive oil

SERVING
- lettuce leaves
- cucumber slice

DIRECTIONS

1. Mix all ingredients in bowl until well incorporated.
2. Preheat a waffle iron and light grease with cooking spray. Cook waffles according to the manufacturer's instructions.
3. Serve with lettuce leaves and cucumber slice between two waffles.
4. Enjoy!

NUTRITIONAL INFORMATION

Calories Per Servings, 260 kcal, 10.27 g Fat, 38.37 g Total Carbs, 7.16 g Protein, 4.7 g Fiber

Buckwheat Porridge

Prep Time   10 min

Servings   4

INGREDIENTS

- 1 cup buckwheat groats
- 3 cups water
- 1 tablespoon walnut butter
- ½ tablespoon salt
- ½ cup soya milk
- 1 teaspoon dates syrup

DIRECTIONS

1. In a saucepan bring water to boil. Add uncooked buckwheat groats. Cover the pot and simmer for 10 minutes (or until water is absorbed).
2. Turn off heat, add the salt, dates syrup and let it sit for 10 more minutes.
3. Top with butter and serve warm in a savory dish, or as a porridge with milk and toppings.

NUTRITIONAL INFORMATION

Calories Per Servings, 188 kcal, 4.6 g Fat, 33.56 g Total Carbs, 5.85 g Protein, 4.2 g Fiber

Toast with Caramelized Apple

Prep Time   10 min

Servings   2

INGREDIENTS

- 2 slice buckwheat bread slices
- 2 oz. chocolate cream
- 1 cup apple
- 2 tbsps. dates syrup
- 1/2 cup water

DIRECTIONS

1. Grill bread for 2 minutes.
2. Heat water in a pan over medium heat.
3. Add dates syrup and apple and cook for 5-8 minutes until apples are soft and caramelize.
4. Spread chocolate cream over the grill bread slice.
5. Sprinkle caramelize apple on top.
6. Serve and enjoy!

NUTRITIONAL INFORMATION

Calories Per Servings, 168 kcal, 7.13 g Fat, 25.45 g Total Carbs, 2.44 g Protein, 2.9 g Fiber

Buckwheat Crepe with Apple

Prep Time   20 min

Servings   4

INGREDIENTS

- 1 cup buckwheat flour
- 2 tbsps. dates syrup
- 1 cup soy milk
- olive oil
- 2 oz. Caramelized apple

DIRECTIONS

1. Mix all ingredients in bowl.
2. Heat oil in pan over medium heat. Once oil is hot pour ¼ cup buckwheat batter and spread evenly.
3. Cook for 2-3 minutes until golden brown.
4. Flip and cook again.
5. Once cooked remove from heat.
6. Wrap with caramelized apple.
7. Serve and enjoy

NUTRITIONAL INFORMATION

Calories Per Servings, 121 kcal, 0.49 g Fat, 32.2 g Total Carbs, 0.85 g Protein, 5.3 g Fiber

Buckwheat & Apple Porridge

Prep Time   20 min

Servings   2

INGREDIENTS
- 1 cup buckwheat groats
- 2 cups soy milk
- pinch of salt
- 1 tsp cinnamon
- 1 sour apple
- Topping
- 1 apple, chopped
- 1 oz. walnuts

DIRECTIONS
1. Bring milk to a boil, season lightly with salt and add buckwheat groats.
2. Add cinnamon to taste, and a grated sour apple.
3. Cook for about 8 minutes, then low the heat and let the buckwheat rest in a covered pot for another 10 minutes.
4. Serve the buckwheat porridge with apple and walnuts topping.
5. Enjoy

NUTRITIONAL INFORMATION

Calories Per Servings, 292 kcal, 10.15 g Fat, 44 g Total Carbs, 10.7 g Protein, 6.2 g Fiber

Acai Berry Smoothie Bowl

Prep Time   5 min

Servings   1

INGREDIENTS

- 1/2 cup walnut milk
- 1 cup acai berry
- 1/4 tsp salt
- Fresh berries for topping

DIRECTIONS

1. Blend milk, berries salt, in a blender and blend on high speed.
2. Pour the smoothie in a bowl.
3. Top with raspberries, blueberries.
4. Serve cool and enjoy!

NUTRITIONAL INFORMATION

Calories Per Servings, 207 kcal, 10.43 g Fat, 27.1 g Total Carbs, 2.42 g Protein, 1.1 g Fiber

Buckwheat Salad Bowl

Prep Time   10 min

Servings   2

INGREDIENTS

- 1 cup buckwheat groats, cooked
- 1 red onion, sliced
- 1bunch parsley leaves
- I bunch arugula leaves.
- 2-3 tomatoes, sliced

DRESSING

- ¼ cup lemon juice
- 1 tbsp. olive oil
- Salt & pepper to taste
- 1 tsp garlic powder.

DIRECTIONS

1. Mix together dressing ingredients in bowl and set aside.
2. Chop veggies and arrange in bowl with cooked buckwheat.
3. Drizzle dressing over veggies.
4. Slightly mix.
5. Serve and enjoy!

NUTRITIONAL INFORMATION

Calories Per Servings, 188 kcal, 0.49 g Fat, 8.37 g Total Carbs, 6.98 g Protein, 5.5 g Fiber

Spinach Avocado Pomegranate Seeds

Prep Time   15 Min

Servings   2

INGREDIENTS

- 1 pack baby spinach
- ½ avocado, thinly sliced
- 4 oz. pomegranate seed

DRESSING

- 1 tbsp. olive oil
- 1 tbsp. lime juice
- 1 pinch salt and pepper

DIRECTIONS

1. Add all veggies in mixing bowl.
2. Mix dressing ingredients in bowl and pour over veggies.
3. Serve cold and enjoy!

NUTRITIONAL INFORMATION

Calories Per Servings, 237 kcal, 15.49 g Fat, 15.49 g Total Carbs, 7.3 g Protein, 9.7 g Fiber

Beetroot Salad with Spinach

Prep Time   15 Min

Servings   2

INGREDIENTS

- 1 pack baby spinach
- 1 beet root, sliced
- 1 oz. walnuts
- 4 oz. cranberries
- 1 oz. feta cheese crumbled

Dressing

- 1 tbsp. sesame oil
- 1 lime juice
- 1 pinch garlic salt

DIRECTIONS

1. Add all veggies in mixing bowl.
2. Mix dressing ingredients in bowl and pour over veggies.
3. Serve cold and enjoy!

NUTRITIONAL INFORMATION

Calories Per Servings, 121 kcal, 0.49 g Fat, 32.2 g Total Carbs, 0.85 g Protein, 5.3 g Fiber

Berries Salad with Spinach

Prep Time   15 Min

Servings   2

INGREDIENTS

1 pack arugula leaves
8 oz. strawberries, sliced
1 oz. walnuts
2 oz. smoked tofu

Dressing
1 tbsp. olive oil
1 lime juice
1 pinch garlic salt

DIRECTIONS

1. Add all veggies in mixing bowl.
2. Mix dressing ingredients in bowl and pour over veggies.
3. Serve cold and enjoy!

NUTRITIONAL INFORMATION

Calories Per Servings, 271 kcal, 22.09 g Fat, 15.48 g Total Carbs, 7.89 g Protein, 4.4 g Fiber

Pomegranate Salad with Spinach

Prep Time   15 Min

Servings   2

INGREDIENTS
- 1 pack baby spinach
- 1 cup pomegranate seeds
- 4-5 lettuce leaves, chopped

Dressing
- 1 tbsp. olive oil
- 1 lime juice
- 1 pinch garlic salt

DIRECTIONS

1. Add all veggies in mixing bowl.
2. Mix dressing ingredients in bowl and pour over veggies.
3. Serve cold and enjoy!

NUTRITIONAL INFORMATION

Calories Per Servings, 237 kcal, 9.35 g Fat, 37.15 g Total Carbs, 8.89 g Protein, 10.8 g Fiber

Hot & Spicy Tofu & Broccoli

Prep Time   20 min

Servings   2

INGREDIENTS
- 8 –12 oz. extra firm tofu
- 2 tbsps. olive oil
- ½ tsp. salt
- 1 tsp. garlic, minced
- 8 oz. broccoli, cut into florets
- 1 tsp. chili sauce and chili flakes
- 1 1/2 Soy Sauce
- 1 tbsp. toasted sesame seeds

DIRECTIONS

1. Heat oil in a large skillet over medium heat.
2. Once oil is hot, add broccoli and cook for 5 minutes.
3. Add salt, pepper and garlic, and cook for 1-2 minutes until the garlic is fragrant.
4. Mix the chili sauce, and soy sauce in a small bowl. Set aside.
5. Fry tofu in same pan for 4-5 minutes.
6. Serve tofu with broccoli.
7. Drizzle sesame seeds on top.
8. Serve and enjoy

NUTRITIONAL INFORMATION

Calories Per Servings, 273 kcal, 22.6 g Fat, 7.19 g Total Carbs, 15.62 g Protein, 4.3 g Fiber

Stir Fried Spinach

Prep Time   20 Min

Servings   2

INGREDIENTS

- 1 lb. spinach, trimmed
- 1 tbsp. paprika
- 1 tbsp. garlic, minced
- Salt and pepper, to taste
- 2-3 whole red pepper
- 2 tbsps. olive oil
- 2 cups vegetable broth

DIRECTIONS

Heat oil in a pan over medium heat.
Once the oil is hot, add garlic and sauté for 1 minute.
Add spinach in the same pan and cook for 4-5 minutes until spinach is welted.
Season with salt, pepper, and whole chili.
Add vegetable broth and cook for 5-10 minutes on medium heat.
Once cooked remove from heat.
Serve hot and enjoy!

NUTRITIONAL INFORMATION

Calories Per Servings, 242 kcal, 8.58 g Fat, 33.74 g Total Carbs, 14.28 g Protein, 9.2 g Fiber

Kale Stew

Prep Time   20 Min

Servings   2

INGREDIENTS
- 1 lb. kale trimmed and cut
- 1 tsp. cumin seeds
- 2 tbsps. dates syrup
- 1 tbsp. paprika
- 1 tbsp. garlic, roughly crushed
- Salt and pepper, to taste
- 2 tbsps. olive oil
- 1 cup vegetable broth

DIRECTIONS
Heat the oil in pan over medium heat.
Once the oil is hot, add garlic and sauté for 2-4 minutes.
Add kale and cook for 4-5 minutes.
Season with salt, pepper, red and dates
Add vegetable broth, garlic and cook for 5-10 minutes on medium heat.
Once cooked remove from heat.
Serve hot and enjoy!

NUTRITIONAL INFORMATION

Calories Per Servings, 161 kcal, 2.9 g Fat, 31.11 g Total Carbs, 11.15 g Protein, 10.6 g Fiber

Stir fry Tofu & Soba Noodles

Prep Time   20 min

Servings   2

INGREDIENTS
8 –12 oz. extra firm tofu
4 oz. soba noodles
2 tbsps. olive oil
½ tsp. salt
1 tsp. garlic, minced
8 oz. broccoli, cut into florets

DIRECTIONS

Boil noodles for 10 minutes in salted water. Drain and set aside.
Heat oil in a large skillet over medium heat.
Add broccoli and cook for 5 minutes until golden brown, over medium heat.
Add salt, pepper and garlic, and cook for another 1-2 minutes until the garlic is fragrant.
Fry tofu in same pan for 4-5 minutes.
For serving add broccoli tofu and noodles in bowl.
Serve and enjoy

NUTRITIONAL INFORMATION

Calories Per Servings, 321 kcal, 7.58 g Fat, 48.27 g Total Carbs, 23.05 g Protein, 3.5 g Fiber

Buckwheat Falafel Bowl

Prep Time   30 Min

Servings   8

INGREDIENTS
FALAFELS
1 onion, roughly chopped
1 tsp. garlic, minced
a large handful parsley
2 cups buckwheat flour
2 tsps. ground cumin
2 tsps. ground coriander
1/8 tsp, pepper & pepper
½ tsp baking powder
Olive oil for deep-frying

TO SERVE

Broccoli florets, stir fried
Brussel sprouts
Cucumber, sliced
Baby Spinach
Arugula leaves
2 lemons, sliced

DIRECTIONS

Add falafel ingredient in food processor and mix well. Add water to make paste

Roll mixture into small falafels the size of walnuts.
Heat oil in pan and cook the falafels, in batches, for 1-2 minutes or until golden.
Remove with a slotted spoon and drain on kitchen paper.
Serve falafel with broccoli, Brussel sprout, cucumber, and veggies. Enjoy!

NUTRITIONAL INFORMATION

Calories Per Servings, 150 kcal, 1.59 g Fat, 30.79 g Total Carbs, 7.52 g Protein, 6 g Fiber

Kale Stew

Prep Time   10 min

Servings   2

INGREDIENTS
I bunch kale, chopped
1 tsp garlic, Minced
3 oz. avocado oil
3 cups vegetables stock
1 tsp Salt
1 tsp Pepper
1 tbsp. Parsley chopped

DIRECTIONS

Sauté the garlic over low heat until they are beginning to turn into brown.
Add kale and rest of ingredients.
Simmer on low to medium heat for 8 Minutes. Once cooked remove from heat.
Stir through the salt, pepper and parsley.
Adjust seasoning to taste.
Enjoy!

NUTRITIONAL INFORMATION

Calories Per Servings, 191 kcal, 8.41 g Fat, 26.19 g Total Carbs, 11.15 g Protein, 11.4 g Fiber

Broccoli Soup

Prep Time   10 min

Servings   2

INGREDIENTS
- 1 medium broccoli florets
- 1 tsp garlic, Minced
- 1 tbsp. olive oil
- 3 cups vegetables stock
- 1 tsp Salt
- 1 tsp Pepper
- 1 tbsp. Parsley chopped

DIRECTIONS

Sauté the broccoli with garlic over low heat until they are beginning to turn into brown.
Add rest of the ingredients.
Simmer on low to medium heat for 8 minutes. Once broccoli is cooked and soft remove from heat.
Carefully blend the soup until no lumps are remaining.
Stir through the salt, pepper and parsley.
Adjust seasoning to taste.
Enjoy!

NUTRITIONAL INFORMATION

Calories Per Servings, 193 kcal, 9.1 g Fat, 23.86 g Total Carbs, 11.31 g Protein, 8.5 g Fiber

Buckwheat Noodles Soup

Prep Time   40 Min

Servings   4

INGREDIENTS

- 1 large onion-diced
- 1 tsp. garlic, minced
- 1–2 tbsps. olive oil
- 1 cup spinach leaves
- 4 cups veggie stock
- 4 cups water
- 6– 8 oz. soba noodles

DIRECTIONS

Sauté the onion for about 2-3 minutes in oil over medium heat, until tender.

Turn heat to medium, add the garlic and continue cook onions until they are deeply golden brown.

Add the veggie stock, water, spinach, noodles and bring to a simmer.

Simmer for 25-30 minutes uncovered on med heat.

Fill bowls with cooked noodles and broth.

Serve immediately.

Enjoy!

NUTRITIONAL INFORMATION

Calories Per Servings, 209 kcal, 1.16 g Fat, 45.53 g Total Carbs, 9.14 g Protein, 2.1 g Fiber

Buckwheat Tortilla

Prep Time   10 min

Servings   6

INGREDIENTS

- 100 grams Buckwheat (soba) flour
- 1 dash Salt
- 1 tbsp. olive oil
- 120 ml to 150 ml Lukewarm water

DIRECTIONS

Combine the buckwheat flour, and salt in a bowl.
Add the water, and form into a ball.
Wrap the dough, and let sit for a while.
Divide the dough into 6 parts
Flatten out into thin, round pancakes, then grill both sides in a frying pan.
Enjoy!

NUTRITIONAL INFORMATION

Calories Per Servings, 76 kcal, 02.77 g Fat, 11.77 g Total Carbs, 2.1 g Protein, 1.7 g Fiber

Sautee Tofu & Kale

Prep Time   10 min

Servings   2

INGREDIENTS

8 –12 oz. extra firm tofu
2 tbsps. olive oil
½ tsp. salt & pepper
1 tsp. garlic, minced
1 bunch kale, chopped

DIRECTIONS

Heat oil in a large skillet over medium heat.
Fry tofu in pan for 4-5 minutes.
Add kale and stir fry for 3-4 minutes until kale is soft.
Add salt, pepper and garlic, and cook for another 1-2 minutes until the garlic is fragrant.
Drizzle sesame seeds on top.
Serve and enjoy!

NUTRITIONAL INFORMATION

Calories Per Servings, 280 kcal, 21.17 g Fat, 12.72 g Total Carbs, 16.17 g Protein, 4.6 g Fiber

Stir Fried Green Beans

Prep Time   10 Min
Servings   2

INGREDIENTS

2 lb. green beans, ends trimmed
1 tbsp. extra-virgin olive oil
2 large garlic cloves, minced
1 tsp. red pepper flakes
1 tbsp. lemon zest
Salt and freshly ground black pepper

DIRECTIONS

Blanch green beans for about 2-4 minutes in a salted boiling water until bright green in color and tender crisp.
Drain and shock in a bowl of ice water to stop from cooking.
Heat a large heavy skillet over medium heat. Add the oil, once oil is hot, add the garlic and red pepper flakes and sauté until fragrant, about 30 seconds.
Add lemon zest and season with salt and pepper.
Serve and enjoy!

NUTRITIONAL INFORMATION

Calories Per Servings, 134 kcal, 5.12 g Fat, 21.21 g Total Carbs, 5.34 g Protein, 8.7 g Fiber

Baked Asparagus

Prep Time   30 Min
Servings   2

INGREDIENTS

1 bunch thin asparagus spears, trimmed
3 tbsps. olive oil
1 clove garlic, minced
1 tsp. oregano
1 tsp. sea salt
½ tsp. ground black pepper
1 tbsp. lemon juice

DIRECTIONS

Preheat an oven to 425 degrees F (220 degrees C).
Place the asparagus into a mixing bowl, and drizzle with the olive oil. Toss to coat the spears, then sprinkle with garlic, salt, oregano, and pepper.

Arrange the asparagus onto a baking sheet in a single layer.
Bake in the preheated oven until just tender, 12 to 15 minutes depending on thickness.
Sprinkle with lemon juice just before serving.

NUTRITIONAL INFORMATION

Calories Per Servings, 234 kcal, 20.59 g Fat, 11.23 g Total Carbs, 5.38 g Protein, 5.2 g Fiber

Broccoli with Olive Tahini

Prep Time   30 Min

Servings   2

INGREDIENTS
1 bunch baby broccoli, trimmed
1 tbsp. olive oil
salt and pepper to taste

OLIVE TAHINI SAUCE
3/4 cup water
3 tbsps. lemon juice
2 tbsps. olive oil
2 garlic cloves
2–3 slices jalapeno
1/4 tsp. salt
¼ cup olives

DIRECTIONS
Brush broccoli with olive oil and sprinkle with salt and pepper.
Place on a parchment lined sheet pan in the oven, to roast until
fork tender about 20-25 minutes.
Meanwhile, place all the tahini ingredients in the blender, and
blend until combined.
Adjust seasoning according to taste.
Arrange the broccoli with tahini sauce in plate.
Drizzle some olive oil and olives on top.
Enjoy!
NUTRITIONAL INFORMATION
Calories Per Servings, 180 kcal, 9.91 g Fat, 15.96 g Total Carbs, 9.4 g
Protein, 7.3 g Fiber

Apple & Walnuts Pie

Prep Time   50 Min

Servings   16

INGREDIENTS

- 8 cups sliced peeled tart apples
- 1 cup dates syrup
- 2 cups walnuts milk
- 2 teaspoons ground cinnamon
- 1 cup walnut butter, softened
- 2 cups buckwheat flour
- 1 cup finely chopped walnuts, divided

DIRECTIONS

Place apples in a greased 13x9-in. baking dish.
Sprinkle with cinnamon. In a bowl, mix flour, milk, syrup and walnuts. in bowl.
Spread mixture over apples. Sprinkle with remaining walnuts.
Bake at 350° for 45-55 minutes or until the apples are tender.
Serve and enjoy!

NUTRITIONAL INFORMATION

Calories Per Servings, 293 kcal, 16.37 g Fat, 36.89 g Total Carbs, 3.89 g Protein, 3.3 g Fiber

Baked Walnut Bars

Prep Time	30 Min

Servings	16

INGREDIENTS
4 tablespoons walnuts butter
3/4 cup buckwheat flour
1/2 teaspoon salt
3/4 teaspoon baking powder
1/8 teaspoon baking soda
1 cup dates chopped
¼ cup dates syrup
1 cup walnuts (chopped)
1 cup dark chocolate melted

DIRECTIONS
Preheat oven to 350 F. Grease and flour an 8-inch square baking pan.
In a medium bowl, mix the flour with salt, baking soda, and baking powder. Whisk or stir to blend thoroughly.
Mix the dates, melted butter, dates and walnuts in blender.
Stir in flour mixture until well blended.
Spoon the thick batter into the prepared baking pan and spread it evenly with a spatula.
Bake in the preheated oven for about 20 to 24 minutes, or until browned and the top has formed a crust.
Drizzle melted chocolate on top. Serve cold and enjoy!
NUTRITIONAL INFORMATION
Calories Per Servings, 170 kcal, 6.57 g Fat, 27.85 g Total Carbs, 2.12 g Protein, 2.1 g Fiber

Coco & Walnuts Milkshake

Prep Time   10 Min

Servings   1

INGREDIENTS

- 1 cup soy milk
- 1 tsp dates syrup
- 1/2 oz. walnuts
- 1 tbsps. coco powder
- 1/2 cup ice cubes

DIRECTIONS
Add all ingredients in high speed blender.
Blend until all ingredients are incorporated.
Serve and enjoy!

NUTRITIONAL INFORMATION
Calories Per Servings, 262 kcal, 17.25 g Fat, 16.09 g Total Carbs, 9.85 g Protein, 1 g Fiber

Walnut Butter Cake

Prep Time   40 Min

Servings   10

INGREDIENTS

- 4 oz. buckwheat flour
- 1 teaspoon baking powder
- 4 oz. walnut butter
- ¼ cup dates syrup
- 1 cup soy milk
- 2 oz. walnut, chopped

DIRECTIONS

Grease cake pan with oil.

Sift the flour and baking powder, set aside.

Add dates syrup sugar and rest of ingredients in it.

Transfer the batter into the greased pan, shake gently to level off the batter.

Bake at a pre-heated oven at 180C (350F) for about 30-35 minutes or until a cake tester inserted into the walnut butter cake comes out clean.

NUTRITIONAL INFORMATION

Calories Per Servings, 195 kcal, 14.06 g Fat, 16.51 g Total Carbs, 3.16 g Protein, 1.5 g Fiber

Walnuts Bits

Prep Time   40 Min

Servings   20

INGREDIENTS
- 1/2 cup walnut butter softened
- 8 oz. walnut cream
- 1/2 cup dates, finely chopped
- cup walnuts, chopped
- 1/2 cup mini chocolate chips
- tbsps.sesame seeds

DIRECTIONS

Line a baking sheet with a silicone mat or parchment paper. Set aside.
In a large bowl, mix all ingredienst except sesame seeds.
Use a cookie scoop to make 20 even bites and place onto prepared cookie sheet.
Roll on sesame seeds.
Place in fridge for 30 minutes - 1 hour, or until firm.
Serve and enjoy!

NUTRITIONAL INFORMATION
Calories Per Servings, 185 kcal, 17.04 g Fat, 7.47 g Total Carbs, 2.92 g Protein, 1.9 g Fiber

Walnuts Muffins

Prep Time   40 Min

Servings   12

INGREDIENTS

- 1/2 cup dates sugar
- 2 cups buckwheat flour
- 2 teaspoons baking powder
- 1/2 teaspoon salt
- 2/3 cup soy milk
- 1/2 cup walnut butter, melted, cooled
- 1 cup dark chocolate, melted
- 1/2 cup California walnuts, chopped

DIRECTIONS

Preheat oven to 400°F. Grease or line 12 large muffin cups.
In large bowl mix, sugars, fnuts, lour, baking powder and salt. In medium bowl combine milk, butter, cgocolate and blend well.
Mix dry ingredients with wet ingredeints.
Pour batter into greased muffin cups.
Bake for 15 to 20 minutes or until cooked.
Serve hot and enjoy!

NUTRITIONAL INFORMATION

Calories Per Servings, 271 kcal, 18.37 g Fat, 23.85 g Total Carbs, 5.51 g Protein, 4.7 g Fiber

Buckwheat Cinnamon Roll

Prep Time   30 Min

Servings   8

INGREDIENTS

- 14-16 oz. buckwheat dough
- 1 cup dates syrup
- 2 tbsps. cinnamon powder,
- 2 tbsps. walnut butter, melted

DIRECTIONS

Preheat oven to 400 degrees F.
Roll dough into a rectangle about 10 X 14 inches.
Mix syrup and cinnamon powder in mixing bowl.
Spread this mixture over rolled dough.
Roll dough in a circle.

Slice dough with knife or pizza cutter into 1-inch pieces. Place rolls on prepared sheets.
Quickly brush butter over rolls.

Bake rolls for about 15 minutes or until lightly brown and rolls are cooked through.

NUTRITIONAL INFORMATION

Calories Per Servings, 170 kcal, 0.41 g Fat, 43.33 g Total Carbs, 1.8 g Protein, 1.4 g Fiber

DOUBLE LAYER NO BAKE CAKE

Prep Time   10 min

Servings   16

INGREDIENTS

- 1 cup walnuts crushed
- 2 cups walnuts cream
- 1 cup chocolate melted
- 4 cups raspberries
- 2 cups walnuts cream

DIRECTIONS

Add walnuts, cream, and chocolate in a bowl and mix well.
Pour mixture in heart shape baking mold and freeze for about 2 hours until set.
Blend raspberries and cream in a blender and pour it over chocolate mixture.
Again freeze for overnight.
Serve and enjoy.

NUTRITIONAL INFORMATION

Calories Per Servings, 274 kcal, 16.59 g Fat, 30.58 g Total Carbs, 4.73 g Protein, 4.3 g Fiber

Fudgy Brownies

Prep Time   40 Min

Servings   12

INGREDIENTS

- 2 cups buckwheat flour
- ¼ cup dates syrup
- 1 tsp. baking powder
- 1 tsp. sea salt
- ½ cup walnut butter, melted
- ½ cup walnut milk
- 1/2 cup cocoa powder

DIRECTIONS
Preheat oven to 350°.
In a large bowl mix dry ingredients and mix wet ingredients in another bowl.
Mix ingredients until well incorporated.
Pour brownies mixture in lined brownies mold.
Bake in preheated oven for about 25-30 minutes until cooked.
Slice it and drizzle chocolate syrup on top.
Serve and enjoy!
NUTRITIONAL INFORMATION
Calories Per serving 156 Cal, Fats 8.97 g, Protein 3.66 g, Total Carbs 19 g, Fiber 3.3 g

Chocolate Pudding With Berries

Prep Time   5 min
Servings   4

INGREDIENTS

- 2 cups walnut milk
- 2 tbsps. chai seeds
- 2 tbsps. coco powder
- 1 tsp dates syrup
- fresh berries, coconut flake for topping

DIRECTIONS

Mix together milk with dates syrup, chia seeds and coco powder in bowl and mix well.
Pour in serving jar and let it stand overnight in fridge.
In morning top pudding with berries.
Serve and enjoy!

NUTRITIONAL INFORMATION

Calories Per serving 136 Cal, Fats 13.05 g, Protein 3.05 g, Total Carbs 4.11 g, Fiber 1.3 g

Chocolate Chip Cookies

Prep Time   30 min
Servings   12

INGREDIENTS

- 1/4 cup olive oil
- 2 tbsps. walnut cream
- 2 cup buckwheat flour
- 1 pinch. sea salt
- 1 tbsps. dates syrup
- 3/4 cup dark chocolate chips

DIRECTIONS
Preheat the oven to 350°.
Mix all ingredients in bowl.
Carefully add chocolate chips into the cookie dough.
Divide the dough into 15 equal balls.
Shape ball and flatten the balls on a greased baking tray.
Bake cookies for about 15-20 minutes in the preheated oven until cooked and golden brown.
Serve and enjoy!
NUTRITIONAL INFORMATION
Calories Per serving 194 Cal, Fats 11.26 g, Protein 3.68 g, Total Carbs 21.08 g, Fiber 3.6 g

WEEK-1 SIRTFOOD MEAL PLAN

MONDAY

BREAKFAST – Spinach Green Juice 181 kcal

LUNCH – Hot & Spicy Tofu & Broccoli 273 kcal

MID DAY SNACK – Berries Green Juice 121 kcal

DINNER – Broccoli Green Juice 187 kcal

TUESDAY

BREAKFAST – Mix Green Juice 146 kcal

LUNCH – Stir Fried Spinach 242 kcal

MID DAY SNACK – Celery Green Juice 118 kcal

DINNER – Kale Green Juice 171 kcal

WEDNESDAY

BREAKFAST – Spinach & Apple Juice 178 kcal

LUNCH – Sautee Tofu & Kale 208 kcal

MID DAY SNACK – Cucumber Green Juice 124 kcal

DINNER – Creamy Spinach Juice 184 kcal

THURSDAY

BREAKFAST - Spinach Green Juice 181 kcal

LUNCH - Pomegranate Salad with Spinach 237 kcal

MID DAY SNACK - Berries Green Juice 121 kcal

DINNER - Kale Stew 191 kcal

FRIDAY

BREAKFAST - Mix Green Juice 146 kcal

LUNCH - Stir fry Tofu & Soba Noodles 321 kcal

MID DAY SNACK - Celery Green Juice 118 kcal

DINNER - Broccoli Soup 193 kcal

SATURDAY

BREAKFAST - Spinach & Apple Juice 178 kcal

LUNCH - Stir Fried Green Beans 134 Kcal

MID DAY SNACK - Cucumber Green Juice 124 kcal

DINNER - Buckwheat Noodles 209 kcal

SUNDAY

BREAKFAST - Spinach Green Juice 181 kcal

LUNCH - Berries Salad with Spinach 271 kcal

MID DAY SNACK - Berries Green Juice 121 kcal

DINNER - Broccoli with Olive Tahini 180kcal

WEEK-2 SIRTFOOD MEAL PLAN

MONDAY

Morning Juice - Berries Green Juice 121 kcal

Breakfast - Apple Porridge 277 kcal

LUNCH - Spinach Avocado Pomegranate Seeds 237 kcal

DINNER - Sautee Tofu & Kale 280 kcal

TUESDAY

Morning Juice - Celery Green Juice 118 kcal

Breakfast - Spinach Omelet 283 kcal

LUNCH - Beetroot Salad with Spinach 121 kcal

DINNER - Stir Fried Green Beans 134 kcal

WEDNESDAY

Morning Juice - Cucumber Green Juice 124 kcal

Breakfast - Tofu & Kale Toast 216 kcal

Sirtfood Diet for Beginners

LUNCH - Berries Salad with Spinach 231 kcal

DINNER - Baked Asparagus 234 kcal

THURSDAY

Morning Juice - Spinach Green Juice 181 kcal

Breakfast - Tofu Scramble 208 kcal

LUNCH - Pomegranate Salad with Spinach 237 kcal

DINNER - Broccoli with Olive Tahini 180 kcal

FRIDAY

Morning Juice - Broccoli Green Juice 187 kcal

Breakfast - Buckwheat Pancakes 197 kcal

LUNCH - Buckwheat Salad Bowl 188 kcal

DINNER - Broccoli Soup 193 kcal

SATURDAY

Morning Juice - Kale Green Juice 171 kcal

Breakfast - Waffle Sandwich 260 kcal

LUNCH - Stir Fried Spinach 242 kcal

DINNER - Buckwheat Noodles 209 kcal

SUNDAY

Morning Juice - Creamy Spinach Juice 184 kcal

Breakfast - Toast with Caramelized Apple 168 kcal

LUNCH - Buckwheat Falafel Bowl 150 kcal

DINNER - Broccoli with Olive Tahini 180kcal

Green Juice with Lime & parsley

Prep Time   10 min

Servings   1

INGREDIENTS

- 1 bunch parsley
- 1 bunch spinach
- 1/2 green apple
- 1 tbsp. lime juice
- 1 tsp. matcha green tea

DIRECTIONS

Extract the juice of spinach, apple and parsley
Pour a Half juice into a glass, then add the matcha, lemon juice
and mix well with fork.
Once the matcha is dissolved add the
remaining of the juice.
Mix well.
Pour some water on top.
Enjoy!

NUTRITIONAL INFORMATION

Calories Per Servings, 151 kcal, 1.97 g Fat, 11.82 g Protein, 29.98 g
Total Carbs, 1.7 g Fiber

Green Juice with Basil & Strawberries

Prep Time   10 min

Servings   1

INGREDIENTS

- 1 bunch basil leaves
- ¼ cup strawberries
- 1/8 tsp. ginger, paste
- half a lemon, juiced
- 1 tsp. matcha green tea

DIRECTIONS

Extract the juice of basil & strawberries
Pour a Half juice into a glass, then add the matcha, lemon juice, ginger paste and mix well with fork.
Once the matcha is dissolved add the
remaining of the juice.
Mix well.
Pour some water on top.
Enjoy!

NUTRITIONAL INFORMATION

Calories Per Servings, 23 kcal, 0.32 g Fat, 1.1 g Protein, 5.11 g Total Carbs, 1.2 g Fiber

Lettuce Green Juice

Prep Time   10 min

Servings   1

INGREDIENTS
- 1 bunch spinach
- 1 bunch lettuce leaves
- ½ green apple
- 1/8 tsp ginger
- half a lemon, juiced
- 1 tsp. matcha green tea

DIRECTIONS

Extract the juice of spinach, apple and lettuce leaves.
Pour a Half juice into a glass, then add the matcha, lemon juice, ginger paste and mix well with fork.
Once the matcha is dissolved add the remaining of the juice.
Mix well.
Pour some water on top.
Enjoy

NUTRITIONAL INFORMATION

Calories Per Servings, 94 kcal, 1.49 g Fat, 10.47 g Protein, 16.19 g Total Carbs, 8.4 g Fiber

Broccoli & Kiwi Juice

Prep Time   10 min

Servings   1

INGREDIENTS

- 2 cups broccoli
- 1 kiwi
- 1 apple
- half a lemon, juiced
- 1 tsp. matcha green tea
- 1 tsp. flaxseeds

DIRECTIONS

Extract the juice of broccoli, apple & kiwi
Pour a Half juice into a glass, then add the matcha, lemon juice
and mix well with fork.
Once the matcha is dissolved add the
remaining of the juice.
Mix well.
Pour some water and flax seeds on top.
Enjoy!

NUTRITIONAL INFORMATION

Calories Per Servings, 136 kcal, 2.19 g Fat, 3.72 g Protein, 30.05 g
Total Carbs, 7.5 g Fiber

Mix Green Juice

Prep Time   10 min

Servings   1

INGREDIENTS

- 1 cucumber
- 1 bunch parsley
- 1 cup rosemary
- 1 cup broccoli
- ½ apple
- half a lemon, juiced
- 1 tsp. matcha green tea

DIRECTIONS

Extract the juice all veggies
Pour a Half juice into a glass, then add the matcha, lemon juice and mix well with fork.
Once the matcha is dissolved add the
remaining of the juice.
Mix well.
Pour some water on top.
Enjoy!

NUTRITIONAL INFORMATION

Calories Per Servings, 121 kcal, 2.32 g Fat, 3.68 g Protein, 25.34 g Total Carbs, 8.6 g Fiber

Basil Juice with Walnuts

Prep Time   10 min

Servings   1

INGREDIENTS

- 2 cups basil leaves
- ½ cup strawberries
- 2 stalk celery with leaves
- ½ cup walnut milk
- 1/8 tsp. ginger, paste
- half a lemon, juiced
- 1 tsp. matcha green tea

DIRECTIONS

Extract the juice of basil, celery, and strawberries
Pour a Half juice into a glass, then add the matcha, lemon juice,
ginger and mix well with fork.
Once the matcha is dissolved add the
remaining of the juice.
Mix well.
Pour milk on top.
Enjoy!

NUTRITIONAL INFORMATION

Calories Per Servings, 106 kcal, 3.06 g Fat, 6.35 g Protein, 15.38 g
Total Carbs, 2.8 g Fiber

Kiwi & Cucumber Juice

Prep Time   10 min

Servings   1

INGREDIENTS

- 1 bunch parsley
- 1 cucumber
- 1 kiwi
- ½ green apple
- half a lemon, juiced
- 1 tsp. matcha green tea

DIRECTIONS

Extract the juice of kiwi, apple, cucumber and parsley.
Pour a Half juice into a glass, then add the matcha, lemon juice and mix well with fork.
Once the matcha is dissolved add the remaining of the juice.
Mix well.
Pour some water on top.
Enjoy!

NUTRITIONAL INFORMATION

Calories Per Servings, 142 kcal, 1.96 g Fat, 6.86 g Protein, 29.96 g Total Carbs, 9.6 g Fiber

Cucumber & Apple Green Juice

Prep Time   10 min

Servings   1

INGREDIENTS

- 1 cucumber
- 1 green apple
- 1 bunch kale
- 1 kiwi
- half a lemon, juiced
- 1 tsp. matcha green tea

DIRECTIONS

Extract the juice of veggies & fruits
Pour a Half juice into a glass, then add the matcha, lemon juice
and mix well with fork.
Once the matcha is dissolved add the
remaining of the juice.
Mix well.
Pour some water on top.
Enjoy!

NUTRITIONAL INFORMATION

Calories Per Servings, 190 kcal, 1.93 g Fat, 7.49 g Protein, 42.86 g
Total Carbs, 10.7 g Fiber

Broccoli & Basil Juice

Prep Time   10 min

Servings   1

INGREDIENTS
- 1 bunch basil
- 1 cucumber
- 1 cup broccoli
- half a medium green apple
- half a lemon, juiced
- 1 tsp. matcha green tea

DIRECTIONS

Extract the juice of basil, apple, cucumber and broccoli.
Pour a Half juice into a glass, then add the matcha, lemon juice
and mix well with fork.
Once the matcha is dissolved add the
remaining of the juice.
Mix well.
Pour some water on top.
Enjoy!

NUTRITIONAL INFORMATION
Calories Per Servings, 102 kcal, 1.19 g Fat, 5.05 g Protein, 21.26 g
Total Carbs, 5.9 g Fiber

Rocket Green Juice

Prep Time   10 min

Servings   1

INGREDIENTS

- 1 bunch rocket leaves
- large stalks green celery, including leaves
- half a medium green apple
- half a lemon, juiced
- 1 tsp. matcha green tea
- 1 tsp. chia seeds

DIRECTIONS

Extract the juice of rocket leaves, apple, and celery
Pour a Half juice into a glass, then add the matcha, lemon juice
and mix well with fork.
Once the matcha is dissolved add the
remaining of the juice.
Mix well.
Pour some water and chia seeds on top.
Enjoy!

NUTRITIONAL INFORMATION

Calories Per Servings, 76 kcal, 0.77 g Fat, 2.55 g Protein, 17.65 g
Total Carbs, 3.8 g Fiber

Walnuts Porridge

Prep Time   20 Min

Servings   2

INGREDIENTS
1 cup soy milk
1 date, chopped
2 tbsps. buckwheat flakes
1 tsp. walnut butter
1 green apple slices
2 oz. pomegranate seeds
1 /2 oz. walnuts

DIRECTIONS

Place the milk and dates in pan over medium heat.
Add the buckwheat flakes, walnuts and cook for 10 minutes.
Once porridge is cooked remove from heat.
Serve with apple slice, pomegranate seeds and walnuts on top.
Enjoy!

NUTRITIONAL INFORMATION

Ca Calories Per Servings, 278 kcal, 11.39 g Fat, 7.28 g Protein,
41.29 g Total Carbs, 5.7 g Fiber

Apple Pancakes

Prep Time   20 min

Servings   4

INGREDIENTS

- 2 apples, puree
- 1 cup, buckwheat flour
- 2 tsp baking powder
- 2 tbsps. dates syrup
- ¼ teaspoon salt
- 1 tbsp. olive oil
- 1 cup blueberries
- 2-3 strawberries, sliced

DIRECTIONS

Mix apple puree, flour, baking powder, dates syrup, and salt to the blender and blend for 2 minutes.

Pour the mixture to a large bowl and fold in half of blueberries.

Heat your skillet over medium heat and grease it with olive oil

Pour ¼ cup pancake batter in skillet and spread it slightly.

Cook pancake for 2-3 minutes per side, until cooked through.

Serve with berries.

Enjoy

NUTRITIONAL INFORMATION

Calories Per Servings, 211 kcal, 4.62 g Fat, 4.43 g Protein, 42.34 g Total Carbs, 6.5 g Fiber

Morning Parfait

Prep Time   10 min

Servings   2

INGREDIENTS
- 1 cup soy yogurt
- 1 cup cranberries
- 1 tbsp. dates syrup
- Mint leaves
- 1 tbsp. walnuts, chopped

DIRECTIONS
Pour 2 tbsps. soy yogurt in serving glass. then layer with cranberries.
Repeat with layer.
Top with dates syrup, mint leaves and walnuts.
Serve cold and enjoy!

NUTRITIONAL INFORMATION
Calories Per Servings, 196 kcal, 2.84 g Fat, 12.48 g Protein, 33.05 g Total Carbs, 1.2 g Fiber

Chocolate Pancakes

Prep Time   20 min

Servings   4

INGREDIENTS

- 1 cup buckwheat flour
- 2 tbsps. cocoa powder
- 1 tsp baking powder
- 2 tbsp. dates syrup
- 3/4 cup soy milk
- 1 tsp. olive oil

DIRECTIONS

Mix buckwheat flour, baking powder, and cocoa powder in mixing bowl.
Add dates syrup, milk and oil and mix well.
Heat nonstick griddle over medium heat, and grease with cooking spray.
Pour ¼ batter in griddle and Let it cook for 2-3 minutes until cooked.
Flip and cook for another 2-3 minutes until cooked through.
Stack the pancakes, drizzle chocolate syrup on top and banana slice.
Enjoy!

NUTRITIONAL INFORMATION

Calories Per Servings, 169 kcal, 3.57 g Fat, 5.23 g Protein, 31.81 g Total Carbs, 3 g Fiber

Spinach Muffins

Prep Time   30 min

Servings   12

INGREDIENTS

2 cups buckwheat flour
¼ cup ground flaxseed
2 tsp. baking powder
½ tsp salt
½ cup soy milk
1 tsp ground cinnamon
½ cup dates syrup
2 cups spinach, chopped
¼ cup walnuts butter

DIRECTIONS
Preheat oven to 375 degrees F.
Mix dry ingredients in bowl and mix well.
Mix wet ingredients in bowl and mix well.
Mix wet ingredients to dry mixture and stir to combine.
Carefully mix chopped spinach in batter.
Pour batter in lined and greased muffin tins.
Bake muffins for about 20-25 minutes or until toothpick comes out clean.
Serve hot with green tea and enjoy!

NUTRITIONAL INFORMATION

Calories Per Servings, 166 kcal, 6.19 g Fat, 3.52 g Protein, 26.94 g Total Carbs, 3.2 g Fiber

Tofu Toast

Prep Time   10 min

Servings   4

INGREDIENTS

- ½ lb. tofu
- 2 onions, sliced
- 1 tsp. garlic, chopped
- 1 tsp of ground turmeric
- 1/8 tsp. pepper & salt
- 2 tbsps. olive oil
- 4 slice buckwheat bread
- chopped parsley for topping

DIRECTIONS

Heat oil in pan over medium heat, once oil is hot, add garlic and fry.
Stir and cook, until it softens.
Add onions and fry on low-medium heat until softened.
Add tofu and mash it with a fork.
Sprinkle with turmeric, salt and pepper and mix well.
Grill buckwheat bread slice on electric grill.
Pour tofu scramble onto warm toast, sprinkle chopped parsley on top.
Serve and enjoy!

NUTRITIONAL INFORMATION
Calories Per Servings, 263 kcal, 18.6 g Fat, 11.78 g Protein, 16.48 g Total Carbs, 4.1 g Fiber

Buckwheat Bread Loaf

Prep Time   60 min

Servings   12

INGREDIENTS

- 1/4 cup melted walnut butter
- 2 apples, puree
- 1/4 cup pure dates syrup
- 2 cups buckwheat flour
- 2 tsps. baking powder

DIRECTIONS

Preheat the oven to 350 degrees F.
Grease 8-inch loaf pan with coconut oil and set aside.
Mix apple, dates syrup and butter in a blender and blend.
Pour the mixture in mix bowl.
Add flour and baking powder in bowl and mix well.
Pour the batter in greased baking loaf pan.
Bake for 40-60 Minutes, or until cooked through.
Allow to cool before cutting.
Enjoy!

NUTRITIONAL INFORMATION

Calories Per Servings, 134 kcal, 4.51 g Fat, 2.65 g Protein, 22.71 g
Total Carbs, 2.7 g Fiber

Broccoli Muffins

Prep Time   40 min

Servings   12

INGREDIENTS

- 2 cups buckwheat flour
- ¾ cup soy milk
- ¼ cup walnut butter
- 1 cup broccoli, roughly chopped
- 4-8 strawberries, sliced
- ¼ cup chopped walnuts
- 1 tsp. cinnamon powder

DIRECTIONS

Mix buckwheat flour, walnuts and cinnamon powder in bowl.

Mix milk, butter, strawberries and broccoli in another bowl,

Gently pour the wet ingredients into the bowl containing the dry ingredients.

Preheat the oven to 200 degrees Celsius.

Line muffin tray with paper liners.

Pour batter into each muffin cup in the tray.

Bake for about 20-25 minutes.

Once cooked remove from oven.

Serve and enjoy!

NUTRITIONAL INFORMATION

Calories Per Servings, 122 kcal, 5.89 g Fat, 3.22 g Protein, 15.89 g Total Carbs, 2.4 g Fiber

Buckwheat Waffles

Prep Time   20 min

Servings   4

INGREDIENTS

- 1 cup buckwheat flour
- ¼ cup walnut butter
- 1/2 cup soy milk
- ¼ tsp. cinnamon powder
- 2 tbsps. dates syrup
- 1 tsp. baking powder

DIRECTIONS

Turn your waffle maker and set it on medium.
Mix together all recipe ingredients in bowl and mix well.
Pour this batter into your waffle maker and cook until the waffle
are cooked and crispy.
Gently remove the waffles from machine.
Serve with walnuts butter on top

NUTRITIONAL INFORMATION

Calories Per Servings, 231 kcal, 13.46 g Fat, 4.96 g Protein, 25.45 g
Total Carbs, 3.4 g Fiber

Eggless Pudding

Prep Time   30 min

Servings   6

INGREDIENTS

8 slice buckwheat bread
1 ½ cups soy milk
2 tbsps. dates syrup
3 tbsps. dates sugar
1 tbsps. walnut butter

DIRECTIONS

Blend bread, milk and dates syrup in blender.
Add sugar with butter in a pan and place it on medium to high heat.
Allow sugar to melt and turn golden.
Transfer the caramel into an oven safe soufflé dish and fill the dish with the bread mixture.
Cover with an aluminum wrap and steam for 25 minutes on low to medium flame.
Once cooked remove from dish.
Refrigerate for at least 2 hours.
Serve and enjoy!

NUTRITIONAL INFORMATION

Calories Per Servings, 239 kcal, 3.17 g Fat, 8.63 g Protein, 48.19 g Total Carbs, 6.1 g Fiber

Turmeric Tea

Prep Time   5 min
Servings   2

INGREDIENTS

2 cups water

1 tsp freshly grated turmeric root

1 tsp freshly grated ginger root

1/2 tsp ground cinnamon

1 tbsp. dates syrup

DIRECTIONS

Place water in a saucepan and heat over medium.
Add the turmeric root, ginger, ground cinnamon and dates syrup and cook for 10 minutes.
Once cooked pour in glass.
Enjoy!

NUTRITIONAL INFORMATION

Calories Per Servings, 38 kcal, 0.09 g Fat, 0.19 g Protein, 10.16 g Total Carbs, 0.7 g Fiber

Green Juicy Salad Bowl

Prep Time   10 min

Servings   2

INGREDIENTS

1 bag, baby spinach

1 cucumber, sliced

16 oz. broccoli, florets

 1 bunch lettuce leaves

4 oz. tofu, fried.

2-3 tomatoes, sliced

DRESSING

2 tbsps. raw apple cider vinegar
1 tbsp. olive
2 garlic cloves, minced
2 tbsps. lemon juice
1 tsp dijon mustard
1/4 tsp salt
2 tbsps. water optional

DIRECTIONS

Mix together dressing ingredients in bowl and set aside.

Fry tofu in pan until brown.

Steam broccoli in microwave with some water.

Chop veggies and arrange in bowl with tofu and broccoli.

Drizzle dressing over veggies.

Slightly mix.

Serve and enjoy!

NUTRITIONAL INFORMATION

Calories Per Servings, 229 kcal, 13.26 g Fat, 17.61 g Protein, 17.93 g Total Carbs, 9 g Fiber

Green Salad with Flaxseed

Prep Time   15 Min

Servings   2

INGREDIENTS

1 pack arugula leaves

1 cucumber sliced

1 red bell pepper, sliced

2-3 tomatoes, sliced

1 tsp. flaxseeds

Dressing

1 tbsp. Italian seasoning
1 tbsp. olive oil
4 tbsps. red wine vinegar
½ tsp salt
¼ tsp ground black pepper
1 tbsp. Dijon mustard

DIRECTIONS
Add all veggies in mixing bowl.
Mix dressing ingredients in bowl and pour over veggies.
Serve cold and enjoy!

NUTRITIONAL INFORMATION
Calories Per Servings, 110 kcal, 8.08 g Fat, 2.29 g Protein, 7.86 g
Total Carbs, 2.5 g Fiber

Beetroot Salad with Spinach

Prep Time   15 Min

Servings   2

INGREDIENTS

1 pack lettuce leaves, chopped

1 cucumber, sliced

8 oz. strawberries, sliced

1 tsp. flaxseeds

Dressing

1 tbsp. olive oil

3/4 cup apple cider vinegar

1/4 cup prepared mustard

1 tbsp. soy sauce

1 tbsp. Splenda

4 cloves garlic, minced

1 tsp. kosher salt

1 tsp. ground black pepper

DIRECTIONS

Cup and slice all veggies and arrange in serving plate.
Mix dressing ingredients in bowl and pour over veggies.
Drizzle flax seeds on top.
Serve cold and enjoy!

NUTRITIONAL INFORMATION

Calories Per Servings, 183 kcal, 10.41 g Fat, 3.61 g Protein, 17.66 g
Total Carbs, 5 g Fiber

Tabbouleh with Lime Dressing

Prep Time   15 Min

Servings   2

INGREDIENTS

1 cucumber, finely chopped

8 oz. spinach, finely chopped

1 red onion finely chopped

1 cup buckwheat groats, cooked

8 oz. parsley, finely chopped

8 oz. strawberries, chopped

Dressing

3 cloves garlic, finely minced

1 ½ tsps. anchovy paste

1 tsp. Worcestershire sauce

2 tbsps. fresh lemon juice

1 ½ tsps. Dijon mustard

Salt and Pepper to taste

DIRECTIONS

Add all chopped veggies and buckwheat in mixing bowl and mix well.
Mix dressing ingredients in bowl and pour over veggies.
Serve cold and enjoy!

NUTRITIONAL INFORMATION

Calories Per Servings, 238 kcal, 2.84 g Fat, 12.96 g Protein, 49.7 g Total Carbs, 12.1 g Fiber

Salad Wrap with Walnut Cream

Prep Time   15 Min

Servings   2

INGREDIENTS

2 buckwheat tortilla

1 cucumber, chopped

4-6 strawberries, chopped

2 lettuce leaves

2 oz. walnut cream

DIRECTIONS

Toss tortilla on griddle until heat up.
Lay tortilla on plate.
Place lettuce leave over it.
Then strawberries and spread walnut cream over it.
Roll tortilla like roll.
Serve with lettuce leaves.
Enjoy!

NUTRITIONAL INFORMATION

Calories Per Servings, 223 kcal, 18.84 g Fat, 5.68 g Protein, 11.71 g
Total Carbs, 3.7 g Fiber

Buffalo Broccoli Bites

Prep Time   40 min

Servings   4

INGREDIENTS
1 head of broccoli, cut into bite sized florets
1 cup buckwheat flour
3/4 cup soy milk
2 tsps. garlic powder
1 1/2 tsps. paprika powder
salt &black pepper
1 tsp. oregano
3/4 cup breadcrumbs
1 cup spicy BBQ sauce

DIRECTIONS

Mix flour, soy milk, water, garlic power, paprika powder, salt, and black pepper in mixing bowl.
Dip the florets into the batter until they are coated well.
Roll florets over the breadcrumbs.
Arrange the florets over baking tray and bake for 25 minutes at 350 °F.
Transfer the cooked broccoli bits to a bowl and coat BBQ sauce over it and bake again for 20 minutes at 350 °F.
Serve immediately and enjoy!

NUTRITIONAL INFORMATION

Calories Per Servings, 161 kcal, 2.77 g Fat, 7.62 g Protein, 30.1 g Total Carbs, 5.5 g Fiber

Creamy Spinach Curry

Prep Time   20 Min

Servings   4

INGREDIENTS

1 lb. spinach, chopped
1 tsp. ginger garlic paste
salt & pepper to taste
1 tsp. paprika powder
1 tsp. cumin seeds
1 tsp red chilli powder
1/2 tsp. turmeric powder
1 tbsp. olive oil
½ cup walnut cream

DIRECTIONS
Heat the oil in a pan over medium heat.
Once oil is hot, add ginger garlic paste and cook for a minute.
Add chopped spinach in pan and cook for 4-5 minutes until spinach is welted.
Add rest of the spices and mix well.
Blender spinach in blender for 1 minutes.
Pour spinach in a pan again, add walnut cream and cook on low heat for about 4-5 minutes.
Once cooked remove from heat, drizzle cream on top.
Enjoy!

NUTRITIONAL INFORMATION
Calories Per Servings, 125 kcal, 9.84 g Fat, 4.51 g Protein, 7.47 g Total Carbs, 3.1 g Fiber

Broccoli Olives Pizza

Prep Time   30 min

Servings   8

INGREDIENTS

1 lb. buckwheat pizza dough

2 tbsp. olive oil

1 bunch broccoli, cut into florets.

1 red onion, sliced

1 tsp minced garlic

salt & pepper to taste

1 oz. BBQ sauce

2 oz. olives

6 oz. tofu, sliced

DIRECTIONS

Heat oil in skillet over medium heat.
Once oil is hot, sauté onion and garlic for 2-3 minutes.
Season with spices and mix well.
Add broccoli in skillet and cook for about 5 minutes.

Preheat oven to 400.
Set buckwheat pizza dough over greased pizza pan.
Cover dough with BBQ sauce. Layer with tofu sliced, cooked broccoli, and broccoli.
Bake for about 10 minutes.
Serve hot and enjoy!

NUTRITIONAL INFORMATION

Calories Per Servings, 296 kcal, 10.7 g Fat, 11.44 g Protein, 44.03 g Total Carbs, 6.9 g Fiber

Spinach Soup

Prep Time   20 Min

Servings   4

INGREDIENTS

1 lb. spinach, chopped

1 tsp. ginger garlic paste

salt & pepper to taste

1 tsp. paprika powder

1 tsp. cumin seeds

1 tsp red chilli powder

1/2 tsp. turmeric powder

1 tbsp. olive oil

3 cups vegetable broth

DIRECTIONS

Heat the oil in a pan over medium heat.
Once oil is hot, add ginger garlic paste and cook for a minute.
Add chopped spinach in pan and cook for 4-5 minutes until
spinach is welted.
Add rest of the spices and mix well.

Blender spinach in blender for 1 minutes.
Pour spinach in a pan again, add broth and cook on low heat for about 4-5 minutes.
Once cooked remove from heat, drizzle cream on top.
Enjoy

NUTRITIONAL INFORMATION

Calories Per Servings, 67 kcal, 4.05 g Fat, 3.7 g Protein, 6.37 g Total Carbs, 3.1 g Fiber

Chilli Tofu

Prep Time   20 Min
Servings   4

INGREDIENTS

8 oz. tofu cut into cubs

1 tbsp. extra-virgin olive oil

2 large garlic cloves, minced

1 tsp. chilli flakes

salt & pepper

1 red chilli, cut into rings

2 tbsps. green onion

Salt and freshly ground black pepper

DIRECTIONS

Heat a large heavy skillet over medium heat. Add the oil, once oil is hot, add the tofu with garlic cook for 5-8 minutes until brown. Season with spices and add red chilli rings.
Drizzle green onion on top.
Serve and enjoy!

NUTRITIONAL INFORMATION

Calories Per Servings, 174 kcal, 12.99 g Fat, 10.02 g Protein, 7.56 g Total Carbs, 2.5 g Fiber

Spicy Spinach Fillet

Prep Time   20 min

Servings   4

INGREDIENTS

1 cup buckwheat Flour

2 cups spinach, chopped

1/2 cup Onions, chopped

1 tsp. red chilli

1/2 cup Kale, chopped

2 tsp. Basil

2 tsp. Oregano

½ cup water

Olive Oil for frying

DIRECTIONS

Mix together all seasonings and vegetables in a large bowl.
Add flour and spicy in same bowl with seasoning and mix
together.
Add water in this mixture and mix.

The mixture should be thick enough to make petties.
Heat oil in skillet over medium heat.
Once oil is hot, cook petties in skillet for about 2-3 minutes.
Flip and cook for another 2-3 minutes until both sides are brown.
Serve with tomatoes slice and enjoy.

NUTRITIONAL INFORMATION

Calories Per Servings, 119 kcal, 1.07 g Fat, 4.75 g Protein, 25.11 g Total Carbs, 4.1 g Fiber

Broccoli Patties

Prep Time   20 min

Servings   4

INGREDIENTS

1 cup buckwheat Flour

1 cup broccoli, chopped

1/2 cup Onions, chopped

1/2 cup Green Peppers, chopped

1/2 cup Kale, chopped

2 tsp. Basil

2 tsp. Oregano

2 tsp. Onion Powder

1/2 tsp. Ginger Powder

½ cup water

Olive Oil for frying

DIRECTIONS

Mix together all seasonings and vegetables in a large bowl.

Add flour and broccoli in same bowl with seasoning and mix together.
Add water in this mixture and mix.
The mixture should be thick enough to make petties.
Heat oil in skillet over medium heat.
Once oil is hot, cook petties in skillet for about 2-3 minutes.
Flip and cook for another 2-3 minutes until both sides are brown.
Serve hot and enjoy!

NUTRITIONAL INFORMATION

Calories Per Servings, 117 kcal, 1.06 g Fat, 4.63 g Protein, 24.85 g Total Carbs, 4.1 g Fiber

Spinach & Tofu Pizza

Prep Time   40 Min

Servings   8

INGREDIENTS

1/2 lb. spinach, trimmed

1 lb. buckwheat pizza dough.

16 oz. tofu, cut into cubes

salt & pepper to taste

1 tsp oregano

1 tsp. chilli powder

1 tbsp. olive oil

1 oz. walnut cream

DIRECTIONS

Preheat the oven to 400°F.

Sautee spinach in a skillet over medium heat, for about 10 minutes until spinach in wilted.

Season with spices and mix well.

Set pizza dough over greased pizza pan.

Spread the walnut cream over pizza dough then spread spinach.

Top with tofu bites.

Bake pizza for 20 about minutes in preheated oven.

Once cooked remove from oven.

Serve and enjoy.

NUTRITIONAL INFORMATION
Calories Per Servings, 254 kcal, 15.93 g Fat, 13.17 g Protein, 19.63 g Total Carbs, 4.8 g Fiber

Broccoli Flatbread Pizza

Prep Time   30 min

Servings   8

INGREDIENTS

1 lb. buckwheat dough

2 tbsp. olive oil

1 bunch broccoli, cut into florets.

1 red onion, sliced

1 tsp minced garlic

salt & pepper to taste

1 oz. walnut cream

DIRECTIONS
Heat oil in skillet over medium heat.
Once oil is hot, sauté onion and garlic for 2-3 minutes.
Season with spices and mix well.
Add broccoli in skillet and cook for about 5 minutes.
Preheat oven to 400.
Set buckwheat dough over greased pizza pan.
Cover dough with walnut cream. Layer with cooked broccoli.
Bake for about 10 minutes.
Serve hot and enjoy!
NUTRITIONAL INFORMATION
Calories Per Servings, 112 kcal, 6.13 g Fat, 3.08 g Protein, 12.97 g
Total Carbs, 2.3 g Fiber

Turmeric Spinach Patties

Prep Time   20 min

Servings   4

INGREDIENTS

1 cup buckwheat Flour

2 cups spinach, chopped

1/2 cup Onions, chopped

1 tbsp. turmeric

1/2 cup Kale, chopped

2 tsp. Basil

2 tsp. Oregano

2 tsp. Onion Powder

1/2 tsp. Ginger Powder

½ cup spring water

olive Oil for frying

DIRECTIONS

Mix together all seasonings and vegetables in a large bowl.

Add flour and spinach in same bowl with seasoning and mix together.
Add water in this mixture and mix.
The mixture should be thick enough to make petties.
Heat oil in skillet over medium heat.
Once oil is hot, cook petties in skillet for about 2-3 minutes.
Flip and cook for another 2-3 minutes until both sides are brown.
Serve hot and enjoy!

NUTRITIONAL INFORMATION
Calories Per Servings, 124 kcal, 1.13 g Fat, 4.86 g Protein, 26.16 g Total Carbs, 4.6 g Fiber

Stir Fried Broccoli & Tofu

Prep Time   20 Min
Servings   4

INGREDIENTS

8 oz. tofu cut into cubes

16 oz. broccoli cut into

1 tbsp. extra-virgin olive oil

2 large garlic cloves, minced

Salt and freshly ground black pepper

2 oz. walnut cream

Spinach leaves

DIRECTIONS
Heat a large heavy skillet over medium heat. Add the oil, once oil is hot, add broccoli with garlic and cook for 4-8 minutes until cooked.
Transfer cooked broccoli in plate.
Add the tofu cook for another 5-8 minutes until brown.
Transfer cooked tofu with broccoli and assemble spinach with them.
Drizzle walnut cream, salt and pepper on top.
Serve and enjoy!

NUTRITIONAL INFORMATION
Calories Per Servings, 287 kcal, 22.75 g Fat, 15.81 g Protein, 11.62 g Total Carbs, 6.3 g Fiber

Wilted Spinach with Onion

Prep Time   40 Min

Servings   2

INGREDIENTS

4 red onions, cut into rings

1/4 cup olive oil

2 1lb. spinach with stems

Salt and freshly ground pepper

DIRECTIONS
Heat oil in large pan over medium heat.
Add the onion rings and cook for about 10-15 minutes over low heat until i=onion is caramelized.
Transfer onion to plate.
Add spinach in same pan and cook for about 5-10 minutes until about to wilted.
 Transfer spinach to plate.
Top with caramelized onion.
Drizzle salt & pepper on top.
Serve and enjoy!

NUTRITIONAL INFORMATION
Calories Per Servings, 300 kcal, 22.79 g Fat, 13.6 g Protein, 18.13 g Total Carbs, 11.1 g Fiber

Broccoli with Garlic sauce

Prep Time   30 Min

Servings   2

INGREDIENTS

1/3 cup minced fresh garlic

2 tablespoons olive oil

1 heat broccoli cut into florets with stems

1 cup vegetable broth

1 tsp. turmeric

salt & pepper to taste

1 tbsp. buckwheat flour

DIRECTIONS

Heat oil in skillet over medium he
Add broccoli florets and cook for 4-5 minutes. Set aside.
Add minced garlic in same skillet and cook for 3 - 5 minutes, until
garlic begins to brown.
Add broth salt & pepper and flour and mix well.
Pour broccoli in skillet again and cook for another 4-5 minutes
until broccoli is soft and sauce is thick.
Serve hot and enjoy!

NUTRITIONAL INFORMATION

Calories Per Servings, 282 kcal, 14.95 g Fat, 11.07 g Protein, 33.39
g Total Carbs, 9.4 g Fiber

Hot & Sour Spinach

Prep Time   40 Min

Servings   2

INGREDIENTS

1 red onion, minced

1/2 cup sherry vinegar

1 thyme sprig

1 tablespoon dates syrup

2 1lb. spinach

3 tablespoons extra-virgin olive oil

Salt and freshly ground pepper

1 cup vegetable broth

DIRECTIONS

Heat oil in pan over medium heat.
Add the onion and cook for about 2-3 minutes over low heat.
Add the vinegar and thyme sprig and bring to a boil.
Simmer over low heat until the vinegar is reduced.
Add dates syrup and mix well.

Add broth in pan, bring to a boil.
Add the spinach and cook until wilted.
Season with salt and pepper and cook for about 5 minutes.
Transfer the spinach to a platter with some broth.
Serve and enjoy!

NUTRITIONAL INFORMATION
Calories Per Servings, 296 kcal, 11.86 g Fat, 15.79 g Protein, 37.91
g Total Carbs, 12.3 g Fiber

Spinach & Tofu Curry

Prep Time   30 Min

Servings   4

INGREDIENTS

2 cups, tofu cubes

2 cups spinach, chopped

2 cloves

1 cardamom

2 tbsps. olive oil

1 green chili, chopped

1 onion, chopped

1 cup walnut milk

½ tsp. ginger-garlic paste

1 tsp. cumin seeds

Salt to taste

DIRECTIONS

Heat oil in a pan over medium heat. once oil is hot, add tofu cubes
and cook for 2-3 minutes.
Transfer fried tofu in plate.

Add the clove, cardamom, cinnamon, and cumin seeds and onion in pan and cook for 2-3 minutes.
Add spinach, milk, salt and ginger-garlic paste.
Stir-fry for 10-15 minutes over medium heat
Add fried tofu stir and combine well.
Once cooked remove from heat.
Serve and enjoy!

NUTRITIONAL INFORMATION
Calories Per Servings, 237 kcal, 11.31 g Fat, 7.34 g Protein, 27.12 g Total Carbs, 1.1 g Fiber

Easy Walnut Milk

Prep Time   5 Min

Servings   4

INGREDIENTS

1 cup walnuts

3 cups filtered water

1/4 tsp cinnamon

DIRECTIONS

Soak walnuts in water for 8 hours or overnight.
 night for at least 8 hours.
In morning strain, the walnuts and place walnuts with filtered water and cinnamon in blender.
Blend for 1-2 minutes.
Strain milk and store in fridge for 3-4 days.
Serve and enjoy!

NUTRITIONAL INFORMATION

Calories Per Servings, 131 kcal, 13.04 g Fat, 3.05 g Protein, 2.88 g Total Carbs, 1.4 g Fiber

Strawberries & Walnut Smoothie

Prep Time   10 Min

Servings   1

INGREDIENTS

1 cup walnuts milk

1 tsp dates syrup

2 oz. strawberries

1 pinch cinnamon

DIRECTIONS

Add all ingredients in high speed blender.
Blend until all ingredients are incorporated.
Serve and enjoy!

NUTRITIONAL INFORMATION

Calories Per Servings, 169 kcal, 13.23 g Fat, 3.43 g Protein, 12.55 g
Total Carbs, 2.5 g Fiber

Walnut Cream

Prep Time   10 Min

Servings   4

INGREDIENTS
2 cups California walnuts
1 cup water
DIRECTIONS
Blend walnuts and water in a high power blender or food
processor until very smooth and light and fluffy.
Store in airtight jar and use in desserts.
Enjoy!
NUTRITIONAL INFORMATION
Calories Per Servings, 262 kcal, 26.08 g Fat, 6.08 g Protein, 5.48 g
Total Carbs, 2.7 g Fiber

Walnut Butter

Prep Time   30 Min
Servings   4

INGREDIENTS

1 1/2 cups walnuts

DIRECTIONS

Roast the walnuts in preheated oven for about 12 minutes until golden brown but not burnt.
Blend the walnut sin food processor for 1-2 minutes.
Scrape and blend for another 1-3 minutes
Store in airtight container and use in desserts.

NUTRITIONAL INFORMATION

Calories Per Servings, 196 kcal, 19.56 g Fat, 4.57 g Protein, 4.11 g Total Carbs, 2 g Fiber

Dark Chocolate Bites

Prep Time   15 min

Servings   8

INGREDIENTS

½ cup walnuts

¼ cup dark chocolate

1 cup Medjool dates, pitted

1 tbsp. cocoa powder

1 tbsp. ground turmeric

1 tbsp. extra virgin olive oil

water

DIRECTIONS
Place the all the ingredients in food processor and mix well.
Add water if required. Mixture should not be sticky.
Form walnut sized balls with your hands and roll over coco
powder.
Freeze balls in freezer.
Once set serve and enjoy!

NUTRITIONAL INFORMATION
Calories Per Servings, 95 kcal, 7.16 g Fat, 1.61 g Protein, 7.37 g
Total Carbs, 1.8 g Fiber

Walnut & Berries Ice-cream

Prep Time   10 min

Servings   2

INGREDIENTS

1 cup walnut cream

1 cup blueberries

DIRECTIONS

Pour walnut cream and half blueberries in blender and mix well.
Pour batter in silicon molds and freeze in freezer for 2- 4 hours
until set and firm.
Serve with fresh berries.
Enjoy!

NUTRITIONAL INFORMATION

Calories per serving 173 Cal, Fats 13.29 g, Protein 3.59 g, Total
Carbs 13.46 g, Fiber 3.1 g

Smoothie with Kiwi

Prep Time   10 min

Servings   2

INGREDIENTS

1 kiwi

1 cup fresh blueberries

2 tbsps. chia seed

1 cup soy milk

¼ cup berries for topping

1 kiwi, slice for topping

DIRECTIONS
Pour kiwi, blueberries in electric high speed blender and blend.
Pour chia seeds in milk and mix well.
Set kiwi slice on the wall of glass and pour milk.
Top with blackberries mixture and fresh blackberries.
Serve cold and enjoy!

NUTRITIONAL INFORMATION
Calories per serving 178 Cal, Fats 2.16 g, Protein 3.78 g, Total
Carbs 38.77 g, Fiber 1.8 g

Blueberries Smoothie

Prep Time   10 min
Servings   1

INGREDIENTS
4-5 strawberries
1/2 cup frozen blueberries
½ cup soy milk
1 cup ice cubes

DIRECTIONS
Mix all the ingredients into a blender, blend until thick and creamy
Pour smoothie in serving glass and top with fresh blueberries and strawberries slice.
Enjoy!

NUTRITIONAL INFORMATION
Calories per serving 113 Cal, Fats 3.1 g, Protein 2.64 g, Total Carbs 20.04 g, Fiber 3.2 g

Chinese Chocolate Truffles

Prep Time   20 Min
Servings   20
INGREDIENTS
16 oz. chocolate
1 cup walnut cream
1 tbsp. Chinese Five Spice Powder
I cup cocoa powder for rolling
DIRECTIONS
Mix together all ingredients in bowl.
Let the mixture sit for 15 minutes.
Freeze the mixture for 2 hours until firm.
Scoop or spoon the mixture into small balls and roll on coco powder.
Refrigerate the rolled truffles for 2 hours.
Serve and enjoy!
NUTRITIONAL INFORMATION
Calories per serving 359 Cal, Fats 26.04 g, Protein 14.5 g, Total Carbs 22.31 g, Fiber 10.1 g

Please let me know if you enjoyed this book with a review, I can't wait to hear news about you!

ABOUT THE AUTHOR

Ashley Gosling is a californian chef and mom based in Los Angeles. After the studies in culinary arts at the San Diego Culinary Institute, she began working in San Diego for a couple years then she had the opportunity to move to Los Angeles to dedicate her career and personal life to her passion for a healthy and sustainable relationship with food.

During the last 15 years she travelled across the world, doing important life experiences especially in Africa, Asia and Europe, visiting the best restaurants and discovering the most unique recipes.
She decided to research and share informations related to healthy food, diets and recipes with as many people as possible, including the most relevant, iconic and promising trends in the culinary and nutrition business.

CPSIA information can be obtained
at www.ICGtesting.com
Printed in the USA
BVHW092054290121
599099BV00009B/2532